Mustapha CHELGHOUM

Hospital Pharmacist's Guide

Mustapha CHELGHOUM

Hospital Pharmacist's Guide

Best practices

ScienciaScripts

Imprint

Cover image: www.ingimage.com

This book is a translation from the original published under ISBN 978-620-6-71242-8.

Publisher:
Sciencia Scripts
is a trademark of
Dodo Books Indian Ocean Ltd. and OmniScriptum S.R.L publishing group

120 High Road, East Finchley, London, N2 9ED, United Kingdom
Str. Armeneasca 28/1, office 1, Chisinau MD-2012, Republic of Moldova, Europe
Printed at: see last page
ISBN: 978-620-8-27414-6

Guide for hospital pharmacists
Good practice

Preamble :

This book is dedicated to ¡exploring good practice in hospital pharmacy, a field where precision, ethics and dedication play a crucial role in the quality of patient care. It is a resource for hospital pharmacists, pharmacy technicians, pharmacy students and other healthcare professionals involved in the management and dispensing of medicines in the hospital environment.

The aim of this book is to provide practical guidance and recommendations based on the latest research and standards of good hospital pharmacy practice. Topics covered range from good manufacturing practice to good traceability practice.

Hospital pharmacy is not just about dispensing medicines; it encompasses a range of essential responsibilities that contribute directly to the safety and efficacy of the treatments administered to patients. Good hospital pharmacy practice requires not only technical expertise, but also the ability to work in a multidisciplinary team, a keen understanding of patient needs and constant adaptation to technological and regulatory developments. The hospital environment is dynamic and requires professionals to be not only providers of care, but also advisors, innovators and leaders in promoting the rational use of medicines.

Table of Contents

Preamble 2
Introduction 7
Chapter 01: Good storage practices 9
Introduction : 9
1. Definitions : 9
2. Good storage practice for pharmaceutical products : 10
Reception and storage : 10
Monitoring stored products : 11
Preserving the quality of pharmaceutical products 12
3. Storage facilities : 13
5. Special storage conditions : 14
Conclusion 16
Bibliography 17
Chapter 2: Good manufacturing practice 18
Introduction 18
1. Definitions 18
2. Evolution of BPP 19
3. Content of good preparation practices : 20
4. Key elements of GMP (ANSM) 21
Quality management 21
Premises 23
Equipment 23
Preparations 23
1. Pharmaceutical raw materials and packaging : 23
2. Preparation operation 24
3.packaging operation : 25
4. Preparation complete : 25
5. Labelling 25

6. Sample library ... 26
7. Control ... 26
How to prevent preparation errors ... 27
Conclusion ... 27
Bibliography ... 28
Chapter 3: Good quality control practices ... 29
Introduction ... 29
1. Regulations and standards ... 29
2. Objective of quality control : ... 29
3. Basic quality control requirements ... 30
4. What to check ... 30
5. Type of quality control ... 31
5.1. Physico-chemical control ... 31
5.1.1. Qualitative and quantitative analysis ... 31
5.1.2. Purity analysis ... 31
5.1.3. Identity analysis ... 31
5.1.4. Stability analysis ... 32
5.1.5. Solubility analysis ... 32
5.2. Pharmaco technical control ... 32
5.2.1. Pharmaco technical control of solid oral forms ... 32
5.2.2. Pharmaco technical control of semi-solid forms ... 36
5.2.3. Example of quality control of an antiseptic ... 37
Conclusion ... 38
References ... 39
Chapter 4: Good practice in traceability ... 40
Introduction : ... 40
1. Definitions : ... 40
2. Pharmaceutical traceability and legislation ... 41
4. Types of tragedy ... 41
5. Objectives for drug traceability ... 41

6. Tragability supports 42
7. Tragability applications for pharmaceutical products 43
8. Tragability means 44
Conclusion 45
Bibliography 46
Chapter 5: Good practice in centralised reconstitution of cytotoxics 47
Introduction 47
1. Definition of Centralised Cytotoxic Reconstitution Units 47
2. Regulations and standards 47
3. Objective 48
4. Benefits of centralisation at pharmacy level 48
5. Design of the CCRU 48
5.1. Types of hoods : 49
5.1.1. Horizontal laminar flow hoods 49
5.1.2. Vertical laminar flow hoods 49
5.1.3. Mixed flow hoods 50
5.1.4. Turbulent flow hoods 50
5.2. Insulators 51
5.2.1 Rigid insulators 51
5.2.2 Flexible insulators 51
5.2.3 Sampling isolators 51
5.3. Cytotoxic contact index (CCI) 51
5.4. Hoods or ZACs 53
5.5. Storage areas in a CCRU 53
5.6. URCC staff 54
6. Anti-cancer drugs circuit in hospital 54
6.1. Receipt of the protocol (prescription) 54
6.2. Pharmaceutical analysis of prescriptions 55
6.3. Production sheet 55

6.4. Manufacture of the preparation 56
6.5. Quality control 56
6.6. Packaging 56
6.7. Routing chemotherapy 57
6.8. Waste management 57
Conclusion 57
Bibliography 58

Introduction

Good hospital pharmacy practice is a fundamental pillar of safe and effective patient care in healthcare organisations. They encompass various critical aspects such as good manufacturing practice (GMP), quality control, drug traceability and specific good practice for the reconstitution of cytotoxic drugs. Each of these elements plays an essential role in preserving the quality of care and preventing medication errors, which can have serious consequences for patient health.

Good Manufacturing Practices are the foundation on which the production of safe and effective medicines is built. In the hospital environment, where medicines are often prepared or adapted to meet the specific needs of patients, GMPs ensure that each product is manufactured in a consistent and controlled manner. This includes validation of processes, qualification of equipment, appropriate training of staff and maintenance of facilities. These practices minimise the risk of cross-contamination, dosing errors and deviations from established standards. Good manufacturing practice is the foundation on which the production of safe and effective medicines is built. In the hospital environment, where medicines are often prepared or customised to meet specific patient needs, GMP ensures that each product is manufactured in a consistent and controlled manner. This includes validation of processes, qualification of equipment, appropriate training of staff and maintenance of facilities. These practices minimise the risk of cross-contamination, dosing errors and deviations from established standards. Quality control is also crucial. It ensures that all medicines dispensed meet the required standards of purity, potency and safety.

In hospital pharmacy, this often involves rigorous testing, including checking the sterility, concentration of active ingredients, and physical and chemical compatibility of preparations. Quality control is essential to detect any deviation that could affect the quality of the medicine and, consequently, patient safety. Drug traceability is another essential component of good hospital pharmacy practice. It makes it possible to track each drug through all the stages of its life cycle, from receipt of the raw materials to administration to the patient. This ability to trace the history, distribution and location of each drug is vital not only to respond effectively in the event of a product recall, but also to investigate adverse reactions and ensure that the right formulations are administered to the right patients. Finally, good reconstitution practices for cytotoxic drugs are of paramount importance in the hospital setting. Cytotoxic drugs, used mainly in the treatment of cancer, are extremely potent and require meticulous handling to avoid exposing staff and other patients to potentially dangerous agents. Standardised reconstitution procedures ensure the safety of those handling these drugs and of the patients who receive them, while maintaining the integrity and efficacy of the treatment.

Commitment to these good practices is therefore essential not only to ensure safety and therapeutic efficacy, but also to enhance the confidence of patients and healthcare professionals in the healthcare system. By developing and rigorously applying these practices, hospital pharmacies play a crucial role in the delivery of high quality, safe and effective healthcare.

Chapter 01: Good storage practices

Introduction :

Managing the storage of medicines is an essential step in the supply chain for healthcare professionals, particularly responsible pharmacists. These professionals must ensure compliance with good practice in the distribution and storage of medicines for human use. The objective of this presentation is to describe guidelines for the storage of medical products that are closely linked to other existing guidelines recommended by the WHO Expert Committee on Specifications for Pharmaceutical Preparations. Organization (2019).

1. Definitions :

Stock: From a physical point of view, stock consists of a set of products deposited and classified in a shop or warehouse. From an economic point of view, stock is a reserve used to regulate supply and demand (Health and Ambulatories 2002).

Good storage practice for pharmaceutical products: Part of quality assurance which ensures that the quality of pharmaceutical products is maintained through adequate control throughout their storage. Organization WH.2019

The legislative basis: As a professional in the field of health, logistics or wholesale, it is important to take into consideration the standards issued by the different actors managing the regulation and the normative production (Board 2006).

Directive 2001/83/EC: This is the main legal instrument for exercising control over the entire distribution chain for medicinal products within Member States, as well as where wholesale operations simultaneously cover several Member States.

European Union guidelines on good distribution practice for medicinal products for human use: They detail good wholesale distribution practice for medicinal products for human use applicable in the EU area in its guidelines of 5 November 2013.

2. Good storage practice for pharmaceutical products :

Reception and storage :

Medicines must be handled and stored in such a way as to avoid spillage, breakage, contamination and mixing. They must not be stored directly on the floor, unless the packaging is designed to allow such storage (as is the case for some medicinal gas cylinders).

If pallets are used, stack the boxes on the pallets.

- at least 10 cm (4 inches) from the ground.
- at least 30 cm (1 foot) from walls and other stacks.
- is no higher than 2.5 m (8 feet, as a general rule).

For all storage :

- Follow the manufacturer's or supplier's instructions on storage procedures and the storage conditions on the labels.
- Place liquid products on the lowest shelves or below other products.
- Store products that need to be kept in controlled areas, maintained at an appropriate temperature.
- Store high-risk/high-value products in appropriate security areas.

■ immediately remove damaged or out-of-date products from usable inventory and dispose of them in accordance with established procedures.

■ Always store products in such a way as to facilitate application of the "first out of date, first out" (FEFO) principle.

■ Arrange the cartons so that the arrows point upwards and the identification labels, use-by dates and production dates are visible.

■ Pharmaceutical depots must have a system for classifying or organising medicines:

- Alphabetical order (by generic name).
- By therapeutic or pharmacological category.
- According to galenic form.
- Depending on the level of the system.
- Depending on frequency of use.
- Randomly, in compartments.
- According to the level of safety and flammability (UNICEF 2003).

Monitoring stored products :

Environmental conditions are important parameters to consider in the storage and distribution of all pharmaceutical products and may need to be monitored as required. Where specific storage conditions are required, environmental loggers or devices should be used to confirm that an acceptable range has been correctly maintained at each stage of the supply chain. Environmental factors to be considered are temperature, light, humidity and cleanliness of the premises.

Temperature is one of the most important conditions to control, the following practices are examples of appropriate measures that should be put in place to ensure environmental control:

■ Recorded temperature monitoring data must be available for review.

■ The equipment used for testing must be checked at appropriate predetermined intervals and the results of these checks must be recorded and retained.

■ It is recommended that temperature monitors be installed in the areas most likely to experience temperature fluctuations (UNICEF and Organization 2003).

Preserving the quality of pharmaceutical products

During storage, different types of products can suffer different types of damage

Type of product	Quality indicators
Liquids	-change in colour -turbidity -presence of sediment -break in cap on bottles -frosted ampoules, bottles or flasks
Photosensitive products	torn or split packaging
Latex products	-dry -friable -cracked
Tablets	change of colour -disaggregated **tablets** -missing tablets - sticky appearance (particularly for coated tablets) - unusual odour
Injectable solutions	**-the** liquid does not form a suspension after shaking
Chemical reagents	- colour change
Tubes	-sticky tube(s) -leaking contents -perforations or holes in the tube

Sterile products	-Torn or split packaging - Missing parts - Broken or bent parts - Moisture inside the packaging - Stained packaging

■ Do not deliver products suspected of being damaged.

■ Report any defects and return faulty products to the supplier.

■ If an inspector visits the school, report any problems (UNICEF and Organization 2003).

3. Storage facilities :

The premises must be designed to ensure that the required storage conditions are maintained. They must be suitably secured, structurally sound and of sufficient capacity to allow safe storage and handling of the medicinal products.

They must have sufficient lighting to allow all operations to be carried out accurately and safely (health and ambulatory care 2002).

5. Special storage conditions :

Pharmaceutical products	Recommendations	Examples
Heat-sensitive medicines	■ Identify which products need to be kept frozen and which need to be stored within a specific temperature range. ■ Keep an eye on the accuracy of the fridge and freezer thermometers. ■ Store medicines in such a way as not to block the circulation of air in the refrigerator. ■ Ensure that refrigerators for storing medicines are reserved for medicines only. ■ Establish a calendar to check the expiry date and rotation of temperature-controlled products (Ziance, Chandler et al. 2009).	*At -20°C for frozen products such as **vaccines**. *Between +2 and +8°C for heat-sensitive products (propofol...)
Photosensitive medicines	■ Hide windows or use curtains. ■ Keep products in cartons. ■ Do not store or package products in direct sunlight. ■ Use opaque plastic or coloured glass bottles for products that require this precaution (UNICEF and Organization 2003).	Furosemide, metronidazole hydrocortisone; vitamins, radio films.
Moisture-sensitive medicines	In a warehouse, the relative humidity must not exceed 60%. ■ All containers must remain closed. ■ They must not be unpacked for too long before distribution. (UNICEF and Organization 2003).	

Medical devices	■ The storage room or area must be able to distinguish between between sterile and non-sterile medical devices. ■Storage must enable the integrity of the medical device to be maintained and contamination of the sterile device to be avoided. ■ Storage must be at an appropriate temperature. (T°C 20°, -2, +5) and humidity (40% to 70%), away from direct sunlight and contamination. ■ The storage material must not generate particles or be a source of alteration to the packaging. ■ Stored DMs must not be piled up or allowed to fall (Ouedraogo, Allou et al. 2020).	*Tubes and drains *Dressing objects *Injection material *ligatures or sutures *Radiological films and accessories. *Small medical equipment.
Flammable products	■ To be stored in a special room, or in a secure cabinet, with sufficient ventilation and retention devices adapted to the quantity stored to prevent and control accidental leaks of polluting liquids (containers and pallets). ■ Isolate from all sources of heat. ■ Fire-fighting equipment must be easily accessible. ■ Do not store in the same areas as medicines. ■ Store in original containers. ■ Store below their flash point. However, it is very important to store them in the coldest place and never in direct sunlight (UNICEF and Organization 2003).	Acetone, anaesthetic ether, alcohols (before dilution) and kerosene.

Corrosive products	■ Always store corrosive substances away from flammable products, preferably in a separate steel cabinet, to prevent leaks. ■ Use suitable industrial gloves and goggles when handling these products (UNICEF and Organization 2003).	Trichloroacetic acid, glacial acetic acid, concentrated ammonia solutions, silver nitrate, sodium nitrate and sodium hydroxide tablets
Medical gases	■ The medical gas premises are secure and inaccessible to the public and unauthorised persons. ■ They enable the bottles to be stored away from bad weather and at a temperature compatible with safety and conservation. ■ The layout of the storage areas allows not only for the separation of different gases and full and empty cylinders, but also for stock rotation (health and ambulatory care 2002).	Medical air. Oxygene - O2. Nitrous oxide - N2O
Limited access products	Identify products at risk of theft or abuse, or with addictive potential, and ensure increased security for these items. These products must be stored in : • A storage room or a separate locked cupboard, or a safe. • A locked metal cage inside the storage room. ■ Only the manager or pharmacist and one other member of staff should be allowed to enter the area where these products are stored (UNICEF and Organization 2003).	Narcotic analgesics (narcotics): MORPHINE, OPIATE PREPARATIONS Other opioids and strong analgesics : CODEINE, BUPRENORPHINE. Psychotropic drugs Other drugs, including antiretrovirals, may need to be stored in a controlled room due to their rarity, cost and high demand.

Conclusion

This directive is intended to apply to all entities involved in any aspect of the storage and distribution of medical products, from the premises of the manufacturer of the medical product to its agent, or the person who dispenses or supplies medical products directly to a patient.

Bibliography

l.Organization WH. Good storage and distribution practices for medical products. WHO Drug Information. 2019;33(2):194-225.

2 Santé Mdl, ambulatoires Ddheds. Guide méthodologique pour la gestion de la pharmacie hospitaliere. 2002.

3. Board IM. Guide to control and monitoring of storage and transportation temperature conditions for medicinal products and active substances. Ireland: Edition Industrial. 2006;3.

4. Guidelines of 5 November 2013 on Good Distribution Practice of medicinal products for human use. Official Journal of the European Union. 2013.

5. Ziance R, Chandler C, Bishara RH. Integration of temperature-controlled requirements into pharmacy practice. Journal of the American Pharmacists Association: JAPhA. 2009;49(3):e61-7; quiz e8-9.

6. UNICEF, Organization WH. Guidelines for the storage of essential medicines and other health commodities. Guidelines for the Storage of Essential Medicines and Other Health Commodities2003. p. 114-.

7 Ouedraogo J, Allou K, El Harti J. Stockage des dispositifs médicaux apres stérilisation: détermination d'une date limite d'utilisation. Le Pharmacien Hospitalier et Clinicien. 2020;55(4):315-21.

Chapter 2: Good manufacturing practice

Introduction

One of the main tasks of hospital pharmacists is to make hospital and magistral preparations in compliance with Good Hospital Preparation Practices. Healthcare professionals and patients have high expectations of the availability of suitable and valid galenic forms that do not exist elsewhere. Controlling their quality is a public health issue. The rigorous application of BPP is essential to the quality control of pharmaceutical preparations.

1. Definitions

Definition of a hospital preparation: this is a medicinal product prepared in a pharmacy for internal use in accordance with the pharmacopoeia under conditions that comply with Good Hospital Preparation Practices, provided that no pharmaceutical speciality is available or suitable in the country. These preparations may only be dispensed on the basis of a medical presentation within the healthcare establishment. (ANSM 2007)

Definition of good hospital compounding practice: GPP is a guide that sets out the principles to be applied to all magistral, hospital and officinal preparations, including preparations of experimental medicinal products and preparations required for biomedical research. This guide therefore applies to all preparations made in hospitals with an authorised IUP or in pharmacies. It is an enforceable standard, the application of which is governed by a publication in the official journal (ANSM 2007).

Magistral preparation: Any medicinal product prepared extemporaneously in a pharmacy in accordance with a medical prescription.

Hospital preparation: any medicinal product prepared on medical prescription and in accordance with the indications of a pharmacopoeia due to the absence of an available or suitable proprietary medicinal product or generic medicinal product, in the pharmacy of a healthcare establishment and intended for dispensing to one or more patients.

Divided officinal product: Any simple drug, chemical product or stable preparation listed in the pharmacopoeia, prepared in advance by a pharmaceutical establishment which divides it up in the same way as a dispensary or hospital pharmacy.

2. Evolution of BPP

Good Preparation Practice 2007

The Good Preparation Practices (GPP) were published in 2007. They apply to pharmacies and pharmacy dispensaries that are responsible for preparing preparations. The BPPs are made up of a first part dealing with general points relating to preparations, a second part containing 2 specific GPs common to pharmacies and IPSs, a third part containing 2 other GPs specific to IPSs and finally a fourth part dedicated to appendices.

Preparation 2023 Good Practices

The decision to rewrite the GPP was based on the age of the current version (dating from 2007) and the report by the Inspectorate General of Social Affairs (IGAS) on the assessment of paediatric parenteral nutrition (PN) practices following the tragedy involving the infants in Chambéry (2013) (Box 2022).

Contaminated bag scandal: In December 2013, three infants hospitalised in the neonatal intensive care unit at Chambéry hospital died suddenly of septic shock within a few days of each other; a fourth was saved at the last minute. All had received parenteral nutrition bags from the same production laboratory. Investigations revealed that bacterial contamination of the TPN bags was a factor in the deaths of the infants. The production of NP bags by this laboratory has since been suspended (Carton 2022).

Updated to 24/10/2023

The latest edition of the guide to good preparation practice (GPP) is now available. Its rules will apply from 20 September 2023, replacing those of 2007.

Compared with the version published in September 2022, the guide incorporates two new guidelines:

- GL3: Preparations required for research involving human subjects, including the preparation of investigational medicinal products;
- and LD4: Preparation of radiopharmaceuticals. This new edition, which supplements the 2022 edition, reinforces the safety requirements for patients exposed to health products, whatever the context of their exposure (ANSM).

3. Content of good preparation practices :

The BPP guide consists of nine general chapters, annexes, guidelines and a glossary:

- The general chapters describe the environmental and operational conditions to be taken into account when making preparations.

- The appendices provide examples to help you implement these best practices.

- The guidelines provide additional information specific to certain types of preparation. When a preparation is covered by several guidelines (GL), they apply simultaneously (for example, the preparation of injectable cytotoxic chemotherapies follows the general chapters, GL1 for the preparation of sterile medicinal products and GL2 for the preparation of medicinal products containing substances that may present a risk to health and the environment) (ANSM 2023).

4. Key elements of GMP (ANSM)

Quality management

The hospital pharmacy quality system depends directly on the hospital quality system and is closely linked to it.

> Organisation: Defined in written procedures:

- The organisation chart
- Who is responsible?
- Who has authority over whom?
- Who depends on whom?
- Staff duties (job descriptions)

> Documentation

- Everything is done in writing;
- The document system must be managed by a procedure;
- The written word is a reliable and accurate means of conveying information;
- They ensure tragability

EXP: Quality manual

- Sets out the establishment's quality policy;
- Describes the quality system;
- Defines quality objectives;
- It must also define: the organisation chart; responsibilities; working relationships between staff; the organisation of the

quality system.

> Non-conformity management

The non-conformity procedure applies when the manufactured product does not meet the requirements (IT IS NON-CONFORMING).

How can non-compliance be managed?

Bring together the people concerned and carry out the following actions:

- Identifying non-compliance ;
- Gather documentation relating to this non-conformity;
- Assessment of non-compliance,
- Proposing corrective action and informing those concerned,
- Drawing up minutes and following up proposed corrective actions.

> Self-assessment

Self-assessment is used to check the establishment's quality system; to ensure that staff use, comply with and apply the various procedures, instructions, etc.; self-assessment must be recorded in minutes or a report.

> Internal audit

The internal audit is an activity of the quality management department, enabling the control of procedures in force to be checked in order to bring about improvement (corrective action) and thus strengthen the establishment's quality system.

> Quality training

- Training and raising staff awareness of quality assurance principles.
- This training must take place initially, i.e. when staff are recruited,

but also as part of ongoing training.

> Staff

- Qualified personnel (must be trained) ;
- The hospital pharmacy is managed by a pharmacist;
- The pharmacist is assisted by :
    - Pharmacy assistants ;
    - Hospital staff ;
    - Administrative staff ;

Premises

- Exclusively reserved for the execution and control of preparations,
- Adapted to the operations to be carried out,
- Easy to clean and disinfect.
- Insulated, well-lit and ventilated
- Sufficient workspace
- Specific rooms for toxic products, narcotics and sterile products
- Smooth, waterproof and crack-free surface

Equipment

- Easy to clean
- Well maintained
- Calibrated and checked regularly

Preparations

1. Raw materials for pharmaceutical use and packaging articles :

- a dated and validated certificate of analysis corresponding to the batch
- If absent: check that the raw material complies with the monograph

- The raw material = a pharmaceutical speciality: no control is required

- The decision of acceptance or refusal is recorded in a register and on the labelling of the container.
- Compliance with storage conditions
- Stock rotation: "first in / first out" and "first to expire / first out".
- Mixing several batches of a PM in the same container is prohibited, as is decanting from the original container.

2. Preparation operation

- Comply with written procedures and instructions;

- Record all data in writing: records are made at the time each action is carried out.

- In the preparation and control area, all containers are identified (name and status of contents) e.g. preparation in progress, preparation awaiting control, production waste).

The following rules apply to all preparations:

- Ensure that equipment, work areas and premises are clean;

- check the status of the equipment: qualification ;

- Check that any PM or AC not used in the preparation and any documents no longer required are removed from the work area;

- ensure that a waste recovery system is available and that it is properly identified;

- carry out the necessary environmental checks;

- check that the equipment used for weighing is fit for purpose and undergoes regular calibration, internally at a defined frequency, and by an approved body at least once a year. Suitable volumetric measuring equipment is also checked using appropriate methods.

3.packaging operation :

-Primary packaging is adapted to the galenic forms it is intended to contain (quantity, quality, dimensions) while avoiding container/content interactions.

- The identity and cleanliness of packaging items are checked.

4. Preparation completed:

-The expiry date for finished preparations is set following bibliographic studies and/or stability tests. Failing this, the expiry date may not exceed one month. This limit may be reduced depending on the stability of the preparation.

5. Labelling

- the name and address of the pharmacy in the establishment or of the pharmacy that prepared the product;

- the designation of the medicinal product: name of the preparation, pharmaceutical form, route of administration and strength in active substance(s); - the prescription number (recorded at the time of dispensing for magistral preparations intended for a single patient),

- expiry date ;

- the specific storage method, if applicable;

- any information to assist in the proper use of the preparation (dosage, method of use, precautions for use, presence of excipients with a known effect, etc.);

- regulatory information in accordance with article

- If justified by particular conditions of use, the preparation is accompanied by instructions for proper use.

6. Sample library

A sample of each batch of finished preparations is kept, unless justified otherwise. The minimum quantity kept must allow at least one complete analysis to be carried out. These samples are kept under the conditions laid down for the preparation for a period at least equal to their expiry date plus one year, unless justified otherwise.

7. Control

Checks are carried out on raw materials, packaging items, finished preparations and environmental monitoring.

The basic requirements are as follows:

- Adapted facilities.

- Qualified staff regularly trained in inspection activities.

- Qualified equipment.

- Validated analysis methods.

Wherever possible, checks are carried out by a different person from the one who prepared the product.

There are different types of control:

- Microbiological controls mentioned in the pharmacopoeia for sterile forms.

- Tests mentioned in the pharmacopoeia monographs for raw materials.

- Galenical controls mentioned in the pharmacopoeia for the different pharmaceutical forms of finished preparations.

- Control made necessary by the nature of the finished preparation, in particular the content of active substance(s).

- Environmental controls (air, surfaces).

How to prevent preparation errors

-Raw materials kept in original packaging

-Preparing and organising the workplace to avoid errors (working from L to R)

Working in a clean manner (to avoid cross-contamination)

-Product labelling and identification at all stages of production

PREPARATION OF INJECTABLE MEDICINES

- Good solvent and dilution

-Working aseptically

-Protecting yourself when handling toxic products

Conclusion

Nevertheless, making pharmaceutical preparations remains a high-risk activity. There are often few French recommendations concerning paediatric use and dosage for certain substances, which means that doctors and pharmacists have to refer to the recommendations in the BPPH guidelines.

Bibliography

1. AN SM. from www.ansm.sante.fr.

2. ANSM (2007). Good preparation practices

3. ANSM (2023). Good preparation practices

4. Carton, C. (2022). "Evolution of good preparation practices: state of the art within 4 preparatories of a university hospital centre."

5. Joradp.dz (2018). "Journal officiel de la république algerienne démocratique et populaire".

Chapter 3: Good quality control practices

Introduction

Hospital preparations are regulated by Algerian and international legislation. They must be prepared in accordance with good preparation practice in order to ensure the quality of the finished product delivered to the patient.

Controls are part of good preparation practice. They ensure that the necessary and appropriate analyses have actually been carried out and that the raw materials, packaging items and preparations made are released for use only if their quality has been judged to be satisfactory.

1. Regulations and standards

In Algeria, drug QC is a legal obligation imposed on all drug manufacturers. Health law no. 18-11 of 2 July 2018 on health stipulates the following in chapter 7, entitled control of pharmaceutical products and medical devices

Art 242: Any pharmaceutical product for use in human medicine, ready for use, and any medical device may not be placed on the market unless it has first been inspected and certified as complying with the registration or approval dossier.

2. Objective of quality control :

Ensuring patient safety: by guaranteeing that the medicines delivered to patients are safe and effective, by checking their quality, identity, purity and concentration.

Regulatory compliance: Hospital pharmacies are subject to strict regulations on the manufacture, control and distribution of medicines.

Quality control processes are designed to ensure that medicines are prepared and dispensed in accordance with current regulations.

Cost optimisation: Quality control can help to reduce costs by minimising losses of raw materials and ensuring the efficiency of production processes.

Patient satisfaction: By guaranteeing the quality and safety of medicines, quality control processes help to improve patient satisfaction and the confidence of healthcare professionals.

3. Basic quality control requirements

□ Adapted facilities,

□ Qualified staff regularly trained in inspection activities,

□ Written procedures are available for sampling, analysis of raw materials and finished preparations,

□ Samples are taken using approved methods,

□ The equipment is qualified and the analysis methods validated,

□ Readings are taken manually and/or using recording equipment,

□ Any batch of preparations may only be released for dispensing by a pharmacist after the pharmacist has ensured that it meets the required specifications,

□ Reference samples of raw materials and finished preparations are kept, except in justified exceptions, in sufficient quantity to allow subsequent control if necessary (in the case of small series).

4. What to check

The quality of a pharmaceutical product is ensured by controls throughout the production chain:

□ Control of raw materials (active substances and excipients) and packaging items.

□ In-process control of semi-finished products (PSO).

□ Inspection of the finished product.

□ These tests must be carried out using validated methods (previously verified pharmacopoeial method or internal method developed and validated by the manufacturer).

5. Type of quality control

- Physico-chemical control ;
- Pharmaco technical control ;
- Microbiological control ;
- Pharmacotoxicological control.

5.1. Physico-chemical control

5.1.1. Qualitative and quantitative analysis

This analysis is used to determine the presence and quantity of different components in the drug. Tests may include chromatography, mass spectrometry, spectrophotometry and other analytical techniques.

5.1.2. Purity analysis

This analysis measures the quantity of foreign substances in the drug. Tests may include gas chromatography (GC), high-performance liquid chromatography (HPLC) and other separation techniques.

5.1.3. Identity analysis

This analysis is used to determine whether the drug is identical to the reference active substance. Tests may include infrared spectroscopy (IR), X-ray diffraction (XRD) and other techniques.

5.1.4. Stability analysis

This analysis measures the drug's ability to maintain its quality and efficacy over time. Tests may include exposing the drug to high temperatures, humidity, light and other environmental factors to assess its stability.

5.1.5. Solubility analysis

This analysis measures the drug's ability to dissolve in a given medium, which can have an impact on its bioavailability and efficacy. Tests may include determination of the octanol/water partition coefficient, measurement of the critical pH and other techniques.

5.2. Pharmaco technical control

Pharmacotechnics is a term that can be broken down into "pharmaceutical techniques", i.e. techniques applied both to the manufacture of medicines and to the control of the pharmaceutical forms obtained.

Unlike physico-chemical and microbiological controls, pharmaco technical controls are specific to the pharmaceutical form being controlled. They make it possible to ensure that this form meets the main characteristics conferred on it by the pharmacopoeia.

Most often, hospital preparations are capsules, powders, syrups or injectable preparations (in the case of reconstitutions of cytotoxic drugs). As more complex pharmaceutical forms such as tablets, ova and soft capsules require industrial equipment, they are not usually prepared in hospital.

5.2.1. Pharmaco technical control of solid oral forms

a) Disaggregation of tablets and capsules

Principle: "This test is designed to determine the ability of tablets or capsules to disintegrate within a prescribed time, in a liquid medium and under well-defined experimental conditions.

The disintegration test is carried out by standardised shaking of the galenic form tested (capsules), in a liquid medium (distilled water) at 37°C, in a tube with a screened bottom.

The test capsules must be completely disintegrated after 30 minutes for the test to be conclusive.

The disintegration test is carried out on 6 units.

If 1 or 2 samples do not disintegrate, repeat the test on 12 additional units.

The test requirements are met if at least 16 of the 18 units tested are disaggregated.

b) Dissolution test for solid forms

The dissolution test is designed to determine the ability of solid oral pharmaceutical forms (tablets and capsules) to allow the active ingredient(s) they contain to pass into solution in a given medium.

The rate of passage into solution is assessed by assaying the active ingredient using chromatographic or spectrophotometric methods in samples taken from the dissolution medium at a given time interval.

Paddle and basket devices are often the most suitable for solid oral forms.

The dissolution test is carried out by plunging a small quantity of the solid form of the drug, such as a pill or tablet, into a container containing a dissolution fluid, (dissolution media: pH: 1.2 (stomach)/ pH: 4.5 (intestine) / pH: 6.8 (resophagus). The container is then placed in a temperature-controlled shaker (37.5°±0.5) to ensure uniform agitation of the dissolution fluid.

Over time, samples of the dissolution fluid are taken at regular intervals and analysed to determine the amount of drug that has dissolved in the fluid. These measurements are used to construct a dissolution curve, which shows the amount of drug dissolving over time.

□ Control of distribution uniformity

When reducing the dose of solid forms (capsules or single-dose powder), the powder must be distributed evenly.

Uniformity of distribution can be controlled in different ways:

- Mass uniformity .
- Uniformity of content.
- Uniformity of single-dose preparations ,

As recommended by the pharmacopoeia.

1) Mass uniformity control

This test is required for capsules (hard capsules), as well as for powders in single-dose containers and tablets.

How it works:

- Individually weigh 20 units taken at random :
- Determine the average mass.

• For single-dose powders: weigh the contents of the 20 units;

• For capsules: Weigh each full capsule.

Without losing any fragments of the capsule shell, open the capsule and empty it as completely as possible, then re-weigh the empty capsule.

Calculate the mass of the contents per difference. Repeat for the remaining 19 capsules.

Interpretation of results:

The individual mass of no more than 2 of the 20 units may deviate from the average mass by a greater percentage than that shown in the table below, but the mass of no unit may deviate by more than twice that percentage.

Average mass of capsules and powders (in single doses)Deviation limits in % of average mass

Less than 300 mg 10

300 mg or more 7.5

Where a uniformity of content test is prescribed for prepared capsules, the uniformity of mass test is not required.

2) Content uniformity control

The content uniformity test applies to capsules / Cp with :

□ The dose of active substance(s) is less than 2 mg,

□ Or in which the active substance represents less than 2% of the total mass.

The content uniformity test is based on the determination of the individual active substance(s) content of the units making up the sample, to check that they are within the established limits in relation to the average content of the sample.

How it works:

- Randomly take 10 units of the preparation to be examined;
- Dose the active substance(s) individually in each of them (appropriate analytical method) ;

Interpretation of results:

- The preparation passes the test if :

The individual content of no more than 1 unit is outside the limits 85 - 115% of the average content and if it is not outside the limits 75 - 125% of the average content.

- The preparation does not pass the test if :

The individual content of more than 3 units is outside the limits of 85 - 115% of the average content, or if the individual content of one or more units is outside the limits of 75 - 125% of the average content.

If the individual content of 2 or 3 units at most differs by 85 - 115% from the average content and if no individual content is outside 75 - 125% :

Randomly take a further 20 units and individually assay the active substance(s) in each of them. The preparation passes the test if the individual contents of no more than 3 of the 30 units are outside the limits of 85 - 115% of the average content and if none of them is outside 75 - 125% of the average content.

5.2.2. Pharmaco technical control of semi-solid forms

1) Homogeneity

- Dosage of P.A
- Macroscopic: spread in a thin layer on a flat surface using a spatula
- Microscopic: control of particle and droplet dispersion

2) Determining consistency :

- Spreading capacity: Measurement of the spreading surface under the action of a given force.
- Extrusion force: Force required to expel a quantity of

ointment from a tube.

- Adhesion power: Measurement of the time required to separate two solid surfaces coated with ointments using a given weight.
- Hardness (consistency control): This involves measuring the penetration of a generally conical mobile into the semi-solid product (Mahleur cone).

3) pH

This is the pH of the aqueous phase, which can be separated more or less easily, depending on the case, by contact, with filter paper, by breaking the emulsion in a water bath, or by centrifugation. For anhydrous ointments, triturate the ointment with distilled water and measure the pH.

4) Sterility

If the ointment is to be applied to open or severely damaged wounds, it should be sterile.

5) Diffusion or bioavailability tests

During the development phase, in vitro tests can be envisaged to see if the ointment does indeed transfer its active ingredient to an aqueous phase. This involves placing a sample of ointment on an aqueous gel (agar or gelatin) and monitoring the diffusion of the active ingredient.

5.2.3. Example of quality control for an antiseptic

1) Features

- Aspect

The appearance is tested visually and directly on the sample in the best light and lighting conditions.

No visible particles

Homogeneity

- Solubility

Be in aqueous or organic solvents (generally water and alcohol)

2) Identification: Colorimetric reaction

3) Dosage: Determination of the quantity of active ingredient by chemical methods

4) Test: pH

Conclusion

Pharmaco-technical tests are essential for assessing the quality of the preparations produced, in order, among other things, to judge their uniformity of distribution and the availability of the active ingredient from these forms.

References

1) Ph. Eur. 8.0 Ed, European Directorate for the Quality of Medicines and Healthcare.

2) Law No. 18-11 of 18 Chaoual 1439 corresponding to 2 July 2018 on health

3) Executive Decree No. 19-379 of 4 Joumada El Oula 1441 corresponding to 31 December 2019

Chapter 4: Good practice in traceability

Introduction :

Tragability is an essential concern in the pharmaceutical field in general and hospital pharmacy in particular. It has become an absolute necessity to ensure patient safety. It involves tracking each drug from the laboratory to the patient to guarantee its quality and integrity.

What motivated the traceability initiative?

□ The emergence of health crises in the 1980s, such as foot-and-mouth disease and mad cow disease. It began with a desire to control the flow of goods through the production chain right up to the delivery of finished products.

□ Between 1984 and 1985, 2,000 haemophiliacs in France contracted the AIDS virus (HIV) through transfusions of contaminated blood. These products were deliberately distributed (Rozenbaum 2008).

1. Definitions :

Tragability: According to ISO 8402:1994, tragability is "the ability to trace the history, use or location of an entity or activity by means of recorded identifications".

Pharmaceutical traceability: This is a regulatory requirement (in Europe) which involves coding each pharmaceutical product to ensure that it can be tracked from the laboratory to the patient.

This codification integrates information such as the product identifier, expiry date, batch number and serial number (Hachachou Nour El HOUDA, 2017).

2. Pharmaceutical traceability and legislation

European regulations impose very strict rules on professionals in the pharmaceutical industry. These regulations are based on two standards:

- GMP: good manufacturing practice for medicinal products,
- GLP: good laboratory practice.

The aim of pharmaceutical traceability is to oblige :

The manufacturer needs to be able to retrace the manufacturing history of a drug, and the operator needs to be able to locate each batch according to its destination (hospital, distributor, medical representatives, etc.).

4. Types of tragedy

- **Upward traceability (tracing):** enables the origin and characteristics of a product to be identified at any point in the chain.
- **Top-down traceability (tracking):** enables raw materials to be traced back to the corresponding finished products and their destinations.
- **Internal traceability**: this refers to the tracking of products within a specific limited area of a global supply chain, such as a hospital pharmacy.
- **External traceability** : External logistics traceability is an identification and recording system that goes beyond the stages a product goes through within the company. It encompasses all links in the supply chain and also includes transit through different countries (when carried out by an external carrier) (Pascal Bonnabry, 2006).

5. Tragability targets for medicines

- Locate a product at any time within a respectable timeframe
- Guaranteeing product quality
- Track the transfer of a product

- Identify the patient to whom a product has been implanted or medication administered
- Protecting patients and healthcare professionals
- Ensure that the drug is accounted for with the recipient
- Ensure product traceability upstream and downstream
- Withdrawing from the market a batch that is defective or at risk of being defective (Hachachou Nour El HOUDA, 2017).

6. Tragability supports

Tragability is organised in two ways: manually and electronically.

-Manual organisation using paper (traditional mode) is the most popular because it is easy to set up and inexpensive, but it is cumbersome to manage, often incomplete and difficult to find information.

-Electronic organisation: this is the most effective, but it is more cumbersome and costly to set up, which means that it is not widely used in hospitals (Pascal Bonnabry, June 2010).

-Tragability media (manual organisation) can be divided into three parts

1. Entry movements (supply)

   - Order book
   - Order form
   - Delivery note
   - The invoice
   - Invoice register

- Receipt form

2. All movements (storage, inventory)
   - Stock sheet / Position sheet / Locker sheet
   - Inventory sheet

3. Exit movements (distribution)
   - Order form (distribution)
   - The order
   - Ledger and special registers
   - The dispensing register

7. Tragability applications for pharmaceutical products

Haemovigilance: Transfusion of LSPs is subject to traceability

Materials vigilance :

• The pharmacist is responsible for ensuring that medical devices are traceable.

• You always need to know which equipment was used for which patient.

• Searches for: nosocomial infections, failure of a medical device and recall of batches by the manufacturer or withdrawal of batches

Biovigilance: this is a monitoring system from the time an organ, tissue or cell is harvested through to the follow-up of transplanted patients. Tragability of harvested and transplanted patients is ensured.

Pharmacovigilance: the pharmacist is responsible for ensuring the traceability of medicines entering and leaving the pharmacy (Brigitte Fumerey, 2007).

Sterilisation: Tragability of sterilisation is an essential safety factor for every practitioner and every patient.

The Medical Devices (MD) to be traced belong to the categories of semi-critical and critical instruments capable of injuring and contaminating human tissue.

Non-critical DM, such as impression trays, labial retractors, photographic mirrors and kneading spatulas, do not need to be traced. This particular category must be disinfected with a detergent-disinfectant or a (thermo)disinfectant washer, but not sterilised.

There are three essential stages in the sterilisation process:

-The creation of a tragability laboratory sheet for each sterilisation, which includes all the autoclave indications, the contents of the sterilised load, the tests carried out and the name and signature of the person carrying out the sterilisation.

-the association of a sterile sachet (and therefore a cycle number) with the patient's file;

-Retention of data on cycles and tests carried out: for a period of 30 years, which is why it is important to scan the test results (staining) stapled to the laboratory form and store them electronically.

8. Tragability means

Marking is a lever for tragability and makes it easier to identify a product.

Tragability information conveyed will be :

- a product identifier

- a unit serial number
- a batch number

- -Linear barcode: Simple, easy to read, but takes up a lot of space if batch number and expiry date.
- -Two-dimensional barcode: A little more complicated to read but allows more information to be stored in a smaller space.
- -RFID (radio frequency identification) chip: Requires a special printer. It can store a lot of information (Pascal Bonnabry, 2006)

Conclusion

The sheer number of tools available to guarantee product traceability can make a pharmacist's work tedious. That's why it's vital to have an excellent command of these tools and to be perfectly organised in their storage, if efficiency is to be improved. The trend is towards computerisation of tools, which makes it easier to fill them in real time. The efficiency of this system is further enhanced when it is coupled with identification equipment such as barcodes or RFID.

Bibliography

1. Rozenbaum, L. (2008). Tragabilité des produits pharmaceutiques en milieu hospitalier, Ed. Techniques Ingénieur.

2. Hachachou Nour El HOUDA: pharmaceutical tragedy 23/12/2017

3. Pascal Bonnabry: Tragability: vigilance and tragability module, 9 March 2006

4. Pascal Bonnabry:Tragability,11th GSASA day,8 and 24 June 2010

5. Laura Di TRAPAN, Sandrine Von Grungun: Stock management tools for pharmaceutical products,6/5/2019

6. Brigitte Fumerey: The duty of tragedy, June 2007

7. https://www.idweblogs.com/hygiene-et-asepsie/la-tracabilite-de-la-sterilisation/

Chapter 5: Good practice in centralised reconstitution of cytotoxics

Introduction

In recent years, cancer chemotherapy has developed considerably. Faced with this increase, the reconstitution of anti-cancer drugs has become a public health issue, and the preparation of anti-cancer drugs by hospitals' central pharmacies has become a matter of course for everyone.

The development of Oncology Pharmacy and the need to strengthen the capacity to prepare cytotoxic drugs by creating CCRUs in health establishments, under the responsibility of a pharmacist.

1. Definition of centralised cytotoxic reconstitution units

More commonly known as the "chemotherapy bubble", it enables all patients' cancer treatments to be prepared in the pharmacy, under the authority of a pharmacist. It provides a controlled environment for the handling, preparation and dispensing of cytotoxic and other hazardous drugs, in compliance with good manufacturing practice standards and regulatory requirements.

2. Regulations and standards

In Algeria, the standards and regulations applicable to URCCs are defined by interministerial order no. 2015-101 of 12 April 2015 relating to the conditions for preparing, holding, dispensing and managing waste cytotoxic medicines and medicines used in targeted cancer therapies.

3. Objective

- Protection of staff, the environment and patient safety through the quality of the preparation administered,
- Ensuring the quality and stability of cytotoxic preparations
- Ensure compliance with regulatory standards and good manufacturing practice
- Optimising the use of resources and skills by streamlining preparation processes
- Ensuring complete traceability of all stages in the preparation and administration of cytotoxics
- Reduce the costs associated with the preparation of cytotoxics by optimising the use of medicines and reducing wastage
- Improve the quality of life of healthcare professionals by limiting their exposure to cytotoxics and reducing the constraints associated with the manual preparation of medicines.

4. Benefits of centralisation at pharmacy level

- Patient safety
- Operator safety
- Clinical follow-up of patients
- Management of leftovers

According to the HAS, "the preparation and reconstitution of cytotoxic drugs must be carried out in a specific unit with an isolator or laminar flow hood under the responsibility of a pharmacist".

5. Design of the URCC

When preparing anti-cancer drugs, it is necessary to protect both the product and the personnel.

Protection is achieved through the use of a ZAC

ZACs will reduce the introduction, multiplication or persistence of contaminating substances.

They are classified into 4 classes:

Class	Environment	Use
A	Review	Preparation of sterile and cytotoxic drugs
B	Controlled	Preparation of non-sterile medicines
C	Limited control	Specific operations (weighing, preparation of raw materials)
D	Occasional inspection	Operations such as labelling or packaging

In a ZAC, specific equipment is available to guarantee the quality and safety conditions required for the preparation of medicines.

5.1. Types of hoods :

5.1.1.Horizontal laminar flow hoods

SMPs are defined as workstations that maintain a sterile environment by providing a filtered airflow through the hood, eliminating airborne particles. This reduces the risk of contamination of prepared medicines and protects staff from handling these potentially hazardous substances.

5.1.2.Vertical laminar flow hoods

They blow clean air vertically downwards over the work area, creating a protected sterile zone for the preparation of sterile medicines. There are two types:

- A (discharge into the room)
- B (discharge outside the room): Protects the preparer from toxicity
- Applications (type IIb)
- Cytostatics.
- Antivirals.
- Other toxic products

5.1.3. Mixed flow hoods

They combine horizontal and vertical laminar flow to create a protected work area for the preparation of sterile and non-sterile drugs.

Maintaining a sterile environment and controlling air contamination is achieved using HEPA filters, which are designed to remove particles from the air by trapping them in a fibre matrix.

GMP recommends the use of type IIB laminar flow hoods.

Type IIA laminar flow hoods can also be used.

5.1.4. Turbulent flow hoods

They blow clean air in all directions to create a protected work area for the preparation of non-sterile drugs.

They blow clean air horizontally over the work area, creating a protective barrier for the products being handled.

However, the personnel working on the sample are not protected, as the blown air is not filtered before entering the work area and can potentially contain contaminants.

5.2. Insulators

It is a closed facility that does not exchange unfiltered air or contaminants with the adjacent environment and is sterile inside.

It creates a watertight physical barrier between the preparation, the manipulator and the environment:

5.2.1 Rigid insulators

These isolators are used for the preparation of highly toxic cytotoxics and require special handling.

Rigid isolators provide a physical barrier between the operator and toxic agents, preventing exposure.

5.2.2 Flexible insulators

These isolators are used for the preparation of less toxic cytotoxic agents, but which still require special handling. Soft isolators are made from flexible materials that adapt to the morphology of the operator and provide a physical barrier between the operator and the toxic agents.

5.2.3 Sampling isolators

These isolators are used to take cytotoxic samples without exposing personnel. Sampling isolators are often used to test air and surface quality in cytotoxic preparation areas.

5.3. Cytotoxic Contact Index (CCI)

C 'is a safety indicator that measures the number of cytotoxic preparations and administrations, as well as working time, using the following formula

ICC = (number of cytotoxic reconstitutions + number of cytotoxic administrations) / (number of working hours)

If ICC < 1 (level I): minimum precautions;
If ICC between 1 and 3 (level II): centralised reconstitution unit desirable
If ICC > 3 (level III): centralised reconstitution unit justified.

There are different formulas for calculating the cytotoxic contact index (CCI), depending on the factors taken into account.

Here are some of the most commonly used formulas:

ICC = (concentration of cytotoxic agent in pg/mL) x (volume of solution prepared in mL) / (contact surface in cm^2 x contact time in hours)

This formula takes into account the concentration of the cytotoxic agent, the volume of solution prepared, the surface area in contact with the solution and the contact time.

ICC = (number of cytotoxic reconstitutions + number of cytotoxic administrations) / (number of working hours)

This formula is used to estimate the level of exposure of workers to cytotoxics over the course of a working day.

ICC = (total quantity of cytotoxics used in mg) / (total weight of exposed workers in kg)

This formula is used to estimate the quantity of cytotoxics used by workers, taking into account their body weight.

5.4. Hoods or ZAC

	Hoods	Insulators
ZAC	B class (SAS in C class)	C or D
Consumables	0.22 pm HEPA filter High cost Constrictive cladding	No dressing or ergonomic constraints
Speaker type	Open enclosure: protection not guaranteed	Enclosure: total protection Preservation of preparations in a sterile atmosphere and sterile packaging of preparations
Number of preparations	< 30day	> 30, day
ICC	ICC between 1 and 3	ICO3
Installation procedures	Draconian procedures	Fewer procedures
Handling	Flexibility of use in an emergency	Emergency problem (biodecontamination takes 10 to 20 minutes)
Coût	1.5 to 3.0 million DA	2 to 3 billion centimes

5.5. Storage areas in a CCRU

They are designed to store the medicines and medical devices needed to prepare chemotherapy and cytotoxics, and are subject to special safety and environmental control requirements to guarantee the quality and stability of the medicines.

They must be located in separate areas dedicated to this function, to avoid any contamination or mixing with other medicines or products.

Storage shelves must be made of stainless steel and easy to clean and disinfect.

5.6. URCC staff

Staff working in a CCRU must be highly qualified and well trained to ensure the safety of patients, staff and the environment. Team members must be made aware of the risks associated with cytotoxic drugs and be trained in the use of personal protective equipment (PPE) and the handling of these products.

All staff handling toxic products must be monitored by the occupational physician at least once a year.

The number of people in the preparation areas is kept to a minimum, access is limited and movement in these areas is controlled.

6. Anti-cancer drugs circuit in hospital

6.1. Receipt of the protocol (prescription)

The protocol describes in detail :

- Patient details: surname, first name, age, weight, height, body surface area.
- The type of pathology and the prior biological work-up.
- The processing cycle number.
- Description of medicines (INN, dosage).
- □ Dosage and methods of administration (central or peripheral route, vehicle, volume, duration).
- Hospital unit concerned.
- Identification of the prescriber.
- Date of prescription and signature.

6.2. Pharmaceutical analysis of prescriptions

- Pharmaceutical patient file.
- Protocol.
- Patient's biological data.
- Indications.
- Checking and recalculating doses.
- Compatibility

6.3. Manufacturing sheet

The patient's identity: name, age, weight, sex and any other information needed to identify the patient.

The identity of the medicine: the name of the medicine, the dose, the route of administration, the dosage and any other information needed to identify the medicine.

Ingredients: the quantity of the various ingredients needed to prepare the drug, including cytotoxics, solvents, diluents and any other necessary components.

Personal protective equipment (PPE): the list of PPE required for preparing the medicinal product, including gloves, gowns, gowns, masks, goggles, etc.

Preparation instructions: detailed instructions for preparing the medicine, including the method of preparation, the steps to be followed, the dosages, and any other information needed to guarantee the quality and safety of the preparation.

Storage conditions: the specific storage conditions for the prepared medicinal product, including temperature, light, humidity and any other conditions necessary to guarantee the stability and quality of the medicinal product.

6.4. Production of the preparation

Reconstitution: Preparation of reconstituted powder in a compatible vehicle,

Dilution: Preparation of the prescribed dose from the mother solution in a bag of saline or glucose solution, depending on physico-chemical compatibility.

Dose-banding (DB): is an Anglo-Saxon concept that was introduced in the late 1990s. It involves simplifying the preparation of cytotoxic drugs by using standardised doses rather than precise doses for each patient. Standardised doses mean that infusions can be manufactured in advance by the pharmacy, which will generate savings not only by using all the bottles of anticancer drugs, but also by allowing unused bags to be returned to stock if a course of treatment is cancelled, subject to compliance with optimum storage conditions.

Good manufacturing practice

6.5. Quality control

Once the preparation has been completed, the pharmacist must carry out a quality control check to ensure that the medicine prepared complies with the planned specifications, particularly in terms of quantity, quality and purity. This control can take various forms, such as visual verification, pH measurement, spectrophotometry, chromatography, etc.

6.6. Packaging

Once quality control is satisfactory, the drug is filled into a suitable sterile container, such as a syringe, vial or bag, following the instructions on the manufacturing sheet. The container is then labelled with all the necessary information, including the name of the drug, dose, route of administration, dosage, date of preparation, shelf life and any other information required.

6.7. Chemotherapy delivery

Only in the "boxes" provided for this purpose (closed containers).

6.8. Waste management

Once the waste has been treated, it must be disposed of in accordance with current regulations, in specific landfill or incineration sites.

Healthcare establishments must ensure that waste is transported and disposed of by specialist companies approved by the competent authorities.

Conclusion

Setting up a Centralised Cytotoxic Drug Reconstitution Unit requires the implementation of rigorous protocols to guarantee the safety of workers and patients, as well as environmental protection. By following good practice, it is possible to create an efficient and safe CCRU for the preparation of cytotoxic drugs.

Bibliography

1. Health Canada (2019). Guidance Document: Good Manufacturing Practices - Guidance on the Preparation of Drug Submission and Applications for Schedule D and Veterinary Drugs. Retrieved from https://www.canada.ca/en/health-canada/services/drugs-health-products/drug- products/applications-submissions/guidance-documents/good-manufacturing-practices/preparation-drug-submission-applications-schedule-d-veterinary- drugs.html#hc1.1.1
2. Agence Frangaise de sécurité sanitaire des produits de santé, Bonnes Pratiques de Preparation, December 2007. https://ansm.sante.fr/documents/reference/bonnes-pratiques-de-preparation, consulted on 18 April 2021.
3. Ministry of Solidarity and Health. Guide méthodologique pour la conception et l'aménagement des unités de reconstitution de cytotoxiques en établissements de santé. 2018.
4. Circular DGS/DHOS/AFSSAPS/DGAS/2005/384 of 30 August 2005 on good practice in the preparation of medicines in pharmacies for internal use
5. French Society of Oncology Pharmacy. Recommendations for good practice in oncology pharmacy. SFPO; 2015.
6. M. Nivault, "Isolateurs et enceintes de confinement", in Les bonnes pratiques de fabrication des médicaments, 5th edition, Lavoisier, 2014, p. 337-341.
7. Principles for the preparation of cytotoxic drugs in a centralised reconstitution unit" by the Société frangaise d'oncologie médicale (SFOM)
8. "Guidance on the Handling of Cytotoxic Drugs and Related Waste" by the National Institute for Occupational Safety and Health

(NIOSH)

9. "Guidelines for the Safe Handling of Hazardous Drugs" by the American Society of Health-System Pharmacists (ASHP)

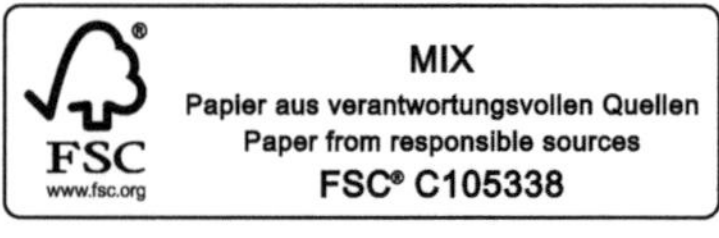

Printed by Books on Demand GmbH, Norderstedt / Germany